# MASTERING TOXIC RELATIONSHIPS

*A Guide To Thriving With A Difficult Partner*

**MELISSA J. POWELL**

## TABLE OF CONTENT

1. Introduction

2. Understanding Toxic Relationships

- Defining Toxicity

- Signs of a Toxic Relationship

- Types of Toxic Behaviors

3. The Cycle of Toxicity

- How Toxic Relationships Develop

- Breaking the Cycle

4. Self-Awareness and Healing

- Recognizing Your Own Patterns

- Self-Care Practices

- Seeking Professional Help

5. Setting Boundaries

- Importance of Boundaries

- Establishing and Enforcing Boundaries

- Communicating Boundaries Effectively

6. Detoxifying Your Relationships

- Identifying Toxic Dynamics

- Strategies for Detoxifying Relationships

- Knowing When to Let Go

7. Building Healthy Relationships

- Characteristics of Healthy Relationships

- Nurturing Positive Connections

- Red Flags to Watch For

8. Maintaining Your Progress

- Staying Mindful of Triggers

- Continuing Self-Work

- Seeking Support Networks

9. Conclusion

# CHAPTER 1

## Introduction

In the labyrinth of our lives, relationships stand as pillars, shaping our experiences, and defining our journeys. Yet, not all relationships are created equal. Some are nurturing, uplifting us to greater heights, while others lurk in the shadows, poisoning our spirits and stunting our growth. This book, "Mastering Toxic Relationships: Break Free, Heal, Thrive," is a beacon of hope amidst the darkness, offering a guiding light for those ensnared in the web of toxicity.

In these pages, you will embark on a transformative journey—a journey of self-discovery, empowerment, and liberation from the chains of toxic relationships. Drawing from psychological insights, personal anecdotes, and real-life examples, this book serves as a roadmap, illuminating the path toward healing and reclaiming your power.

Whether you're entangled in a toxic partnership, navigating tumultuous familial dynamics, or grappling with toxic friendships, this book provides the tools, strategies, and wisdom to navigate these treacherous waters. From recognizing toxic patterns to setting boundaries, from fostering self-love to cultivating healthy relationships, each chapter serves as a stepping stone toward freedom and fulfillment.

But this journey is not merely about survival; it's about thriving. It's about transcending the scars of the past and stepping into the radiant authenticity of your being. It's about reclaiming your voice, your agency, and your worth. It's about transforming wounds into wisdom, chaos into clarity, and despair into resilience.

So, if you find yourself shackled by the chains of toxicity, if you yearn for liberation and restoration, if you dare to reclaim your sovereignty and rewrite your story—then this book is for you. Together, let us embark on a journey of healing, growth, and empowerment. Together, let us master toxic relationships and emerge victorious, radiant, and free.

# CHAPTER 2

Understanding Toxic Relationships

Defining Toxicity

Signs of a Toxic Relationship

Types of Toxic Behaviors


In a world where relationships are celebrated as the cornerstone of human connection, it's essential to understand the darker nuances that can lurk beneath the surface. Toxic relationships, shrouded in manipulation, deceit, and emotional turmoil, can wreak havoc on one's mental and physical well-being. To traverse these treacherous waters, one must first unravel the intricate layers of toxicity that can entangle even the strongest of bonds.

# Defining Toxicity

At its core, toxicity in relationships stems from behaviors and dynamics that are harmful, manipulative, or emotionally draining. It transcends mere disagreements or conflicts, delving into patterns of control, abuse, and imbalance of power. Toxicity can manifest in various forms, from subtle manipulation to outright aggression, leaving individuals feeling trapped and powerless.

## Signs of a Toxic Relationship

Recognizing the signs of toxicity is paramount in safeguarding one's emotional health. It often begins with a sense of unease or discomfort, gradually escalating into a pervasive feeling of dread or anxiety. Common indicators include:

**1. Lack of Trust**: Constant suspicion, jealousy, and dishonesty erode the foundation of trust within the relationship.

**2. Constant Criticism**: Constructive feedback is replaced with relentless criticism, leading to feelings of inadequacy and self-doubt.

**3. Isolation**: Toxic partners may seek to isolate their significant other from friends, family, and support networks, fostering dependence and control.

**4. Gaslighting**: Manipulative tactics such as gaslighting, where one denies or distorts reality, can leave victims questioning their sanity and perception of events.

**5. Cycle of Abuse:** In abusive relationships, cycles of tension, explosion, and remorse perpetuate a cycle of violence and manipulation.

## Types of Toxic Behaviors

Toxic behaviors manifest in myriad ways, each leaving its own trail of destruction in its wake. Understanding these behaviors is crucial in identifying and addressing toxicity within relationships:

**1. Narcissism:** Characterized by a sense of entitlement, lack of empathy, and manipulation, narcissistic partners prioritize their own needs and desires above all else.

**2. Codependency:** Codependent relationships thrive on unhealthy patterns of enabling, rescuing, and sacrificing one's own needs for the sake of the other.

**3. Control and Manipulation:** Manipulative tactics, such as guilt-tripping, gaslighting, and emotional blackmail, serve to control and dominate the partner, eroding their autonomy and self-esteem.

**4. Emotional Abuse:** Emotional abuse encompasses a range of behaviors, including verbal attacks, intimidation, and invalidation, aimed at undermining the victim's sense of self-worth and agency.

**5.  Addiction and Dependency:** Relationships marred by addiction or dependency, whether substance abuse or behavioral addictions, perpetuate a cycle of dysfunction and instability.

In conclusion, understanding toxic relationships requires a keen awareness of the subtle yet insidious dynamics that underpin them. By recognizing the signs of toxicity and familiarizing oneself with the various forms it can take, individuals can empower themselves to break free from harmful patterns and cultivate healthier, more fulfilling connections.

# CHAPTER 3

The Cycle of Toxicity

How Toxic Relationships Develop

Breaking the Cycle

In the intricate tapestry of human relationships, there exists a phenomenon that often goes unnoticed until it's too late: the cycle of toxicity. This destructive pattern can permeate any relationship, leaving emotional scars and wreaking havoc on individuals' lives. But fear not, for within the depths of this darkness lies the potential for transformation and growth.  Below, I will explain how toxic relationships developes and how to break free from them.

## The Anatomy of Toxicity

To understand how toxic relationships develop, we must first dissect the anatomy of toxicity itself. From subtle manipulation to outright abuse, toxicity can manifest in various forms, each with its own set of consequences. Through real-life examples and psychological insights, we'll explore into the underlying dynamics that fuel these destructive patterns, shedding light on the intricate interplay of power, control, and dependency.

## The Seeds of Toxicity

Like weeds in a garden, toxic relationships often begin with seemingly innocuous seeds that take root and flourish over time. Whether it's a lack of communication, unresolved conflicts, or unchecked insecurities, these initial cracks in the foundation can quickly escalate into full-blown toxicity if left unaddressed. By identifying these early warning signs and addressing them head-on, we can prevent the cycle of toxicity from taking hold.

The Spiral of Dysfunction

As toxicity takes root, it begins to spiral out of control, creating a cycle of dysfunction that feeds upon itself. From escalating conflicts to cyclical patterns of abuse and apology, the dynamics of toxic relationships can trap individuals in a never-ending loop of pain and despair. Through case studies and expert analysis, we'll explore how this downward spiral unfolds, shining a light on the insidious mechanisms that keep individuals trapped in its grip.

## Breaking the Chains

But amidst the darkness, there is always hope. In this chapter, we'll explore strategies for breaking free from the cycle of toxicity and reclaiming our autonomy and self-worth. From setting boundaries to seeking support, there are countless ways to dismantle the chains that bind us and forge a path towards healing and transformation. Drawing upon the wisdom of survivors and therapists alike, we'll chart a course towards liberation, empowering readers to take back control of their lives and rewrite their own narratives.

## Cultivating Healthy Relationships

Breaking free from toxicity is only the first step on the journey towards a happier, healthier future. In this final chapter, we'll explore strategies for cultivating and maintaining healthy relationships that nourish the soul and foster growth and fulfillment. From effective communication to mutual respect and empathy, building strong foundations based on trust and understanding is key to breaking free from the cycle of toxicity once and for all.

## Finally:

As we reach the end of our journey, it's important to remember that healing is a process, not a destination. While the cycle of toxicity may leave scars that linger, it does not define who we are or dictate our future. By understanding the dynamics at play, learning from our experiences, and embracing the power of resilience, we can break free from the chains of toxicity and embrace a future filled with love, joy, and possibility. So let us take this knowledge and forge ahead, for the path to healing begins with a single step.

# CHAPTER 4

Self-Awareness and Healing

Recognizing Your Own Patterns

Self-Care Practices

Seeking Professional Help


Understanding oneself is like a
tricky journey, where we figure out

who we are bit by bit. It's like a puzzle, and being self-aware helps us solve it. We start by noticing our habits, thoughts, and feelings that make us who we are.

Self-awareness is like being the boss of our own thoughts and feelings. It helps us understand ourselves better. It's like a guide that helps us explore our thoughts and feelings, even the ones we might not like. By doing this, we can understand why we do the things we do and let go of stuff that holds us back.

But self-awareness isn't just about noticing stuff; it's also about making changes. Once we know our habits and feelings, we can take care of ourselves better. It's like taking care of a garden, where we plant seeds of self-love and acceptance and make ourselves feel better.

Taking care of ourselves is like a special routine that shows we're important. It can be simple things like going for a walk or doing meditation. Each time we do something nice for ourselves, it's like saying we're worth it.

Sometimes, though, we need more than just self-care. When things get tough, it's okay to ask for help from people who know how to help us. Getting help isn't a weakness; it's a sign that we're brave enough to get the support we need.

Therapy or counseling can be really helpful when we're going through tough times. It's like having a map and someone to guide us through our feelings. They listen to us and help us find our way back to feeling better.

In life, understanding ourselves and healing are like important parts of a big picture. They help us become stronger and happier. They give us the power to move past our problems and build a better future. With each step, we become more confident, find our purpose, and realize how important we are.

# CHAPTER 5

Setting Boundaries

Importance of Boundaries

Establishing and Enforcing Boundaries

Communicating Boundaries Effectively

Setting boundaries is crucial for maintaining healthy relationships, promoting self-respect, and fostering personal growth. Boundaries define the limits of acceptable behavior, both for oneself and others, creating a framework for interaction that promotes emotional and psychological well-being. *Below, we'll explore the importance of boundaries, how to establish and enforce them, and the art of communicating boundaries effectively.*

## **<u>Importance of Boundaries:</u>**

Boundaries serve as guidelines for acceptable behavior, allowing individuals to protect their physical, emotional, and mental space. They help to establish a sense of self-respect and self-worth by signaling what is and isn't acceptable treatment. Without boundaries, individuals may find themselves in situations where their needs are ignored, leading to resentment, frustration, and even exploitation.

Healthy boundaries also contribute to the maintenance of relationships. By clearly defining what is acceptable and what is not, boundaries prevent misunderstandings and conflicts. They foster mutual respect and understanding, as each person's limits are acknowledged and respected.

Furthermore, boundaries are essential for personal growth and development. They enable individuals to prioritize their own needs and goals, rather than constantly accommodating others at the expense of their well-being. By setting boundaries, individuals can carve out space for self-care, pursuing their passions, and nurturing their mental health.

## Establishing and Enforcing Boundaries:

Establishing boundaries requires self-awareness and introspection. Individuals must identify their own needs, values, and limits to determine what constitutes acceptable behavior in various contexts. This process involves reflecting on past experiences, recognizing patterns of discomfort or resentment, and identifying areas where boundaries are needed.

Once boundaries are established, enforcing them becomes essential. This involves clearly communicating boundaries to others and assertively upholding them when they are crossed. Enforcing boundaries may involve saying "no" to requests that violate one's limits, setting consequences for boundary violations, or even distancing oneself from individuals who consistently disregard boundaries.

However, enforcing boundaries can be challenging, especially in situations where there is pressure to prioritize others' needs over one's own. It requires courage, self-confidence, and assertiveness to stand firm in the face of resistance or manipulation. Nevertheless, the long-term benefits of maintaining boundaries far outweigh the temporary discomfort of confrontation.

## Communicating Boundaries Effectively:

Effective communication is key to establishing and maintaining boundaries. It involves clearly articulating one's needs, limits, and expectations in a respectful and assertive manner. ***Here are some*** *strategies for communicating boundaries effectively:*

**1.  Be Direct and Specific:** Clearly state what behavior is acceptable and what is not. Avoid ambiguity or hints, as this can lead to misunderstandings.

**2.  Use "I" Statements:** Frame boundaries in terms of your own feelings and needs, rather than criticizing or blaming others. *For example, instead of saying, "You always interrupt me," say, "I feel disrespected when I'm interrupted."*

**3.  Set Consequences:** Clearly communicate the consequences of violating boundaries. This might involve withdrawing from the situation, ending the conversation, or taking other action to protect your well-being.

**4. Be Consistent:** Consistently enforce boundaries to demonstrate their importance and maintain credibility. Inconsistency can lead to confusion and undermine the effectiveness of boundaries.

**5. Listen Actively:** Encourage open dialogue and be receptive to others' perspectives, while still maintaining your own boundaries. Effective communication is a two-way street, and listening is just as important as speaking.

**6. Seek Support:** If you're struggling to communicate or enforce boundaries, seek support from trusted friends, family members, or professionals. They can offer guidance, validation, and encouragement as you navigate boundary-setting.

**Finally:,** setting boundaries is essential for maintaining healthy relationships, promoting self-respect, and fostering personal growth. By establishing clear boundaries, enforcing them assertively, and communicating them effectively, individuals can create a framework for interaction that prioritizes their well-being and fosters mutual respect and understanding.

# CHAPTER 6

Detoxifying Your Relationships

Identifying Toxic Dynamics

## Detoxifying Your Relationships:

In our lives, relationships play a vital role in our happiness and well-being. However, just like our bodies need detoxification from harmful substances, our relationships sometimes require detoxification from toxic dynamics. Let's explore how you can detoxify your relationships effectively.

## 1. Identifying Toxic Dynamics:

Before you can detoxify your relationships, it's crucial to recognize toxic dynamics. These can include:

*Manipulation:* When one person tries to control or manipulate the other for their own benefit.

*Constant Criticism:* Excessive criticism can erode self-esteem and create a negative atmosphere.

*Lack of Trust:* Without trust, a relationship can't thrive, and suspicion can poison interactions.

*Unhealthy Boundaries:* When boundaries are crossed or disregarded, it can lead to resentment and conflict.

*Communication Issues:* Poor communication, such as yelling or stonewalling, can breed misunderstanding and frustration.

## 2. Strategies for Detoxifying Relationships:

Once you've identified toxic dynamics, it's time to implement strategies to detoxify your relationships:

*Open Communication:* Foster honest and open communication to address issues and concerns calmly and constructively.

*Set Boundaries:* Establish clear boundaries and communicate them respectfully. This ensures that both parties' needs and limits are respected.

*Practice Empathy:* Seek to understand the other person's perspective and feelings, fostering empathy and compassion.

*Seek Support:* Sometimes, professional help or counseling can provide valuable insights and tools for improving relationships.

*Focus on Positivity:* Cultivate positivity by expressing gratitude, celebrating achievements, and focusing on the good aspects of the relationship.

### 3. Knowing When to Let Go:

Despite our best efforts, some relationships may be beyond repair. Knowing when to let go is essential for your well-being:

*Evaluate the Relationship:* Reflect on whether the relationship brings more harm than good and if efforts to improve it have been futile.

*Listen to Your Instincts:* Trust your instincts and feelings. If you consistently feel drained, unhappy, or unsafe in the relationship, it may be time to let go.

*Prioritize Self-Care:* Recognize that letting go of toxic relationships is an act of self-care and self-respect.

*Seek Closure:* If possible, seek closure by communicating your decision respectfully and honestly, allowing both parties to move forward.

*Detoxifying your relationships* requires courage, self-awareness, and sometimes difficult decisions. By identifying toxic dynamics, implementing healthy strategies, and knowing when to let go, you can cultivate healthier, more fulfilling relationships in your life.

# CHAPTER 7

## Building Healthy Relationships

- Characteristics of Healthy Relationships

- Nurturing Positive Connections

- Red Flags to Watch For

## Building Healthy Relationships

Relationships are the cornerstone of human interaction, offering companionship, support, and fulfillment. Building healthy relationships requires understanding the key characteristics, nurturing positive connections, and being aware of red flags that can signal potential problems. In this comprehensive guide, we'll explore each of these aspects in detail, providing insights and strategies for cultivating strong, meaningful connections with others.

## Characteristics of Healthy Relationships

Healthy relationships are characterized by several key traits that contribute to their strength and longevity. These characteristics include:

**1. Communication:** Effective communication is essential for any healthy relationship. This involves openly expressing thoughts, feelings, and needs while also listening actively to your partner. Good communication fosters understanding, trust, and intimacy.

**2. *Trust:*** Trust forms the foundation of healthy relationships. It's built through honesty, reliability, and consistency in actions over time. Trust allows individuals to feel secure and confident in their relationship, knowing they can depend on their partner.

**3. *Respect:*** Respect is fundamental in healthy relationships, encompassing appreciation, consideration, and valuing each other's opinions and boundaries. Respectful behavior fosters mutual admiration and creates a positive environment where both partners feel valued and understood.

**4. Empathy:** Empathy involves understanding and sharing the feelings of others. In healthy relationships, partners are empathetic towards each other's experiences, showing compassion and support during both joyful and challenging times.

**5. Equality:** Healthy relationships are characterized by equality, where both partners contribute equally to decision-making, responsibilities, and compromises. Each person's needs and desires are respected and considered with fairness and balance.

**6. Support:** Supportive relationships provide encouragement, comfort, and assistance during life's ups and downs. Partners actively support each other's goals, dreams, and aspirations, fostering a sense of teamwork and mutual growth.

**7. *Independence:*** While healthy relationships involve interdependence and connection, they also respect individual autonomy and independence. Partners maintain separate identities, interests, and friendships, allowing for personal growth and fulfillment outside of the relationship.

**8. *Conflict Resolution:*** Conflicts are inevitable in any relationship, but healthy couples approach them constructively, seeking resolution through communication, compromise, and understanding.

They work together to address issues and find mutually satisfactory solutions.

## Nurturing Positive Connections

Building and maintaining positive connections in relationships requires ongoing effort and attention. Here are some strategies for nurturing healthy relationships:

*1. Prioritize Quality Time:* Spend meaningful time together, engaging in activities that strengthen your bond and deepen your connection. This could include sharing hobbies, going on dates, or simply enjoying each other's company.

*2. Practice Active Listening:* Listen attentively to your partner's thoughts, feelings, and concerns without interrupting or judging.

Validate their experiences and demonstrate empathy by acknowledging their perspective.

**3. *Show Appreciation:*** Express gratitude and appreciation for your partner regularly, acknowledging their efforts, qualities, and contributions to the relationship. Small gestures of kindness and recognition can go a long way in fostering positivity and mutual admiration.

**4. *Cultivate Trust:*** Be honest, reliable, and transparent in your actions, earning your partner's trust through consistency and integrity. Avoid behaviors that erode trust, such as dishonesty, secrecy, or betrayal.

**5. *Communicate Effectively:*** Foster open and honest

communication by expressing your thoughts, feelings, and needs clearly and respectfully. Listen actively to your partner's perspective and seek to understand before being understood.

**6. *Maintain Boundaries:*** Respect each other's boundaries and autonomy, understanding that healthy relationships require space for individual growth and self-expression. Communicate openly about boundaries and honor each other's limits and preferences.

**7. *Resolve Conflict Constructively:*** Approach conflicts as opportunities for growth and understanding, rather than as threats to the relationship. Practice active listening, empathy, and compromise to find mutually satisfactory solutions.

**8. Foster Intimacy:** Cultivate emotional, physical, and sexual intimacy in your relationship, prioritizing affection, closeness, and vulnerability. Share your thoughts, feelings, and desires openly, deepening your emotional connection over time.

## Red Flags to Watch For

While every relationship encounters challenges, certain behaviors and dynamics may indicate underlying issues that warrant attention. Here are some red flags to watch for in relationships:

**1. Lack of Communication:** Communication breakdowns or

avoidance can signal underlying issues that need to be addressed. If one or both partners are unwilling or unable to communicate openly and honestly, it can strain the relationship.

**2. Distrust or Betrayal:** A lack of trust or repeated instances of betrayal, such as lying, cheating, or deception, erode the foundation of the relationship. Trust is essential for a healthy connection, and persistent distrust can lead to resentment and insecurity.

**3. Disrespectful Behavior:** Verbal, emotional, or physical abuse, as well as disrespectful attitudes or actions, are serious red flags in any relationship. Such behavior undermines mutual respect and can cause lasting harm to both partners.

**_4. Control or Manipulation:_**
Attempts to control or manipulate your partner's thoughts, feelings, or actions are signs of unhealthy power dynamics. Healthy relationships are built on mutual respect and autonomy, not coercion or manipulation.

5. Lack of Support: If your partner consistently undermines your goals, dismisses your feelings, or fails to offer support during challenging times, it may indicate a lack of investment in the relationship. Supportive partnerships are built on encouragement, empathy, and collaboration.

**6. Isolation:** Isolating tactics, such as limiting your contact with friends and family or controlling your social interactions, are warning signs of abusive behavior. Healthy relationships respect each other's social connections and encourage independence outside of the partnership.

**7. Unresolved Conflict:** Persistent unresolved conflicts or patterns of escalating arguments can indicate underlying issues that need to be addressed. Avoiding or minimizing conflicts without seeking resolution can lead to resentment and distance in the relationship.

**8. Emotional Distance:** Emotional distance or detachment from your partner, characterized by a lack of intimacy, affection, or connection, may signal deeper issues in the relationship. It's essential to address underlying concerns and work towards re-establishing emotional closeness.

In conclusion, building healthy relationships requires understanding and embodying key characteristics such as communication, trust, respect, and empathy. Nurturing positive connections involves prioritizing quality time, effective communication, and mutual support, while being mindful of red flags such as lack of communication, distrust, disrespect, and control. By cultivating these qualities and addressing potential issues proactively, individuals can foster strong, fulfilling relationships that stand the test of time.

# CHAPTER 8

Maintaining Your Progress

Staying Mindful of Triggers

Continuing Self-Work

***Maintaining progress*** in any aspect of life requires dedication, awareness, and ongoing effort. Whether you're striving for personal growth, professional success, or health and wellness, it's essential to establish strategies to sustain your achievements over time. Here's a detailed look at three key components for maintaining progress: staying mindful of triggers, continuing self-work, and seeking support networks.

## Staying Mindful of Triggers:

Progress often involves breaking old habits or patterns that may have held you back in the past. However, these habits can resurface when faced with triggers – situations, emotions, or environments that prompt a return to previous behaviors. Staying mindful of these triggers is crucial for maintaining progress.

One way to identify triggers is through self-reflection and introspection. Take the time to explore your thoughts, feelings, and behaviors to uncover patterns and recognize what tends to derail your progress. Once you've identified your triggers, develop strategies to cope with them effectively.

*For example,* if stress is a trigger for overeating, you might implement stress-reduction techniques such as mindfulness meditation or deep breathing exercises. If social situations trigger anxiety or self-doubt, practice assertiveness skills or seek out supportive friends or family members who can help bolster your confidence.

By remaining vigilant and proactive in managing triggers, you can minimize their impact and maintain forward momentum in your journey of progress.

**Continuing Self-Work:**

Personal growth is an ongoing process that requires continuous self-reflection and improvement. Even when you've made significant strides, there's always room for further development and refinement. Continuing self-work is essential for sustaining progress over the long term.

Self-work encompasses various activities aimed at enhancing self-awareness, self-esteem, and overall well-being. This may include practices such as journaling, therapy, meditation, or engaging in activities that promote personal growth and fulfillment.

Regular self-assessment is also crucial for monitoring your progress and identifying areas that may need attention or improvement. Set aside time for introspection and self-evaluation, asking yourself questions like: What are my strengths and weaknesses? What have I learned from past experiences? What are my goals for the future, and how can I work towards them?

By committing to ongoing self-work, you can deepen your understanding of yourself, cultivate resilience, and continue to evolve in positive ways.

**Seeking Support Networks:**

Maintaining progress is often easier with the support of others. Surrounding yourself with a supportive network of friends, family, mentors, or like-minded individuals can provide encouragement, accountability, and valuable insights.

Seek out individuals who share your goals or who have successfully navigated similar challenges. Connect with them for guidance, advice, or simply a listening ear during times of struggle or uncertainty.

Support networks can also offer practical assistance in the form of resources, referrals, or opportunities for collaboration. Whether it's joining a support group, participating in community events, or seeking out online forums and social networks, finding a supportive community can be instrumental in sustaining progress.

Additionally, don't hesitate to lean on your support network when facing setbacks or obstacles. Remember that progress is not always linear, and setbacks are a natural part of the journey. Having a supportive community to turn to during difficult times can help you stay resilient and stay on course towards your goals.

In summary, maintaining progress requires a combination of awareness, effort, and support. By staying mindful of triggers, continuing self-work, and seeking support networks, you can cultivate resilience and sustain your achievements over the long term.

# CHAPTER 9

Conclusion

In the journey through the intricate web of toxic relationships, we've explored into the depths of human emotions, vulnerabilities, and the power dynamics that shape our interactions. From recognizing the warning signs to implementing effective strategies for self-care and boundary-setting, the path to mastering toxic relationships is one fraught with challenges but ripe with opportunities for growth and transformation.

As we reach the conclusion of this book, it's essential to reflect on the profound insights gained and the invaluable lessons learned. We've unearthed the roots of toxicity, dissected its various manifestations, and armed ourselves with the tools necessary to navigate these treacherous waters with grace and resilience.

*But mastering toxic relationships isn't just about avoiding or escaping them—it's about reclaiming our power, honoring our worth, and cultivating healthy connections that nourish our souls. It's about recognizing that we are deserving of love, respect, and kindness, and refusing to settle for anything less.*

As we bid farewell to the pages of this book, let us carry forward the wisdom gained and the courage instilled within us. Let us embrace the journey of self-discovery and self-love, knowing that we possess the strength to transcend the toxicity that once held us captive.

*May this book serve as a guiding light for those navigating the murky waters of toxic relationships, illuminating the path toward healing, liberation, and authentic connection. And may each reader find solace in the knowledge that they are not alone—that there is hope, and there is a way forward.*

*In the end, mastering toxic relationships is not just about surviving—it's about thriving. It's about reclaiming our power, rewriting our narratives, and forging ahead on a path of liberation and wholeness.* So let us embark on this journey together, with courage in our hearts and a steadfast determination to create the relationships we deserve. For in mastering toxic relationships, we ultimately master ourselves.

www.ingramcontent.com/pod-product-compliance
Lightning Source LLC
Chambersburg PA
CBHW081810250726
48653CB00010B/3881